HERPES: Lysine Foods to Eat to Manage Herpes Outbreaks

With Recipes!

Kayleigh Lee

© Copyright 2023 - All rights reserved.

The content contained within this book may not be reproduced, duplicated or transmitted without direct written permission from the author or the publisher.

Under no circumstances will any blame or legal responsibility be held against the publisher, or author, for any damages, reparation, or monetary loss due to the information contained within this book, either directly or indirectly.

Legal Notice:

This book is copyright protected. It is only for personal use. You cannot amend, distribute, sell, use, quote or paraphrase any part, or the content within this book, without the consent of the author or publisher.

Disclaimer Notice:

Please note the information contained within this document is for educational and entertainment purposes only. All effort has been executed to present accurate, up to date, reliable, complete information. However, no warranties of any kind are declared or implied. Readers acknowledge that the author is not engaged in the rendering of legal, financial, medical or professional advice. The content within this book has been derived from various sources. Please consult a licensed professional before attempting any techniques outlined in this book.

By reading this document, the reader agrees that under no circumstances is the author responsible for any direct or indirect losses incurred as a result of the use of the information contained within this document, including, but not limited to, errors, omissions, or inaccuracies.

Table of Contents

Table of Contents	3
The Role of Amino Acids in Herpes Replication	12
The Importance of Lysine and Arginine in Herpes Replication	12
How Lysine Can Help Prevent Herpes Outbreaks	12
Scientific Evidence for Lysine and Herpes	12
The Effect of Lysine on Herpes Outbreaks	14
The Significance of the Lysine/Arginine Ratio in Foods	14
Tips for Maintaining a Lysine-Rich Diet	14
Recommended Daily Intake of Lysine Through Supplementation	14
How to Use this Guide	16
Foods with the Highest Lysine to Arginine Ratio	18
Margarine	18
Yogurt fruit low fat	18
Yogurt plain	18
Yogurt plain skim	18
Yogurt plain low fat	18
Cheese swiss	18
Cheese gruyere 6+ months aged	18
Cheese American spread	18
Cheese edam	18
Cheese gouda Dutch	18
Whey sweet dry	19
Cheese blue	19
Cheese provolone 2-3 months	19
Papaya fruit called Pawpaw in Australia	19
Cheese brie	19
Cheese camermbert	19
Cheese parmesan	19
Cheese parmesan grated	19
Cheese goat brown	19
Cheese brick	19
Milk goat's	19
Cheese muenster orange with white	20
Beets	20
Cheese limburger stinky-cheese	20
Cheese port du salut	20
Cheese tilsit yellow semi-soft	20

Cheese American processed	20
Cheese swiss processed	20
Cheese mozzarella	20
Cheese mozzarella grated	20
Cream cheese	20
Cheese neufchatel soft white French	20
Butter common	21
Cheese colby	21
Cheese monterey Jack semi-hard	21
Buttermilk	21
Cheese cheddar	21
Cheese cheshire	21
Half & half cream	21
Milk skim	21
Sherbet powder	21
Ice cream	21
Milk condensed	21
Milk dry instant non fat	21
Milk dry non fat	22
Milk evaporated	22
Milk evaporated skim	22
Milk iced	22
Milk low fat	22
Milk whole	22
Milk whole dry	22
Whipping cream heavy	22
Whipping cream light	22
Ice cream rich	22
Mango fruit	22
Whipped cream pressurized	22
Apricots fruit	23
Apples	23
Coffee cream	23
Cheese ricotta	23
Cheese ricotta part skim	23
Milk chocolate flavour	23
Pears dried	23
Eggnog milk drink	23
Apple sauce unsweetened	23
Crabapple fruit slices	23
Loquat fruit	23

Apples dried	23
Pears fruit	24
Milk carob flavour	24
Apricots dried	24
Cottage cheese creamed	24
Cottage cheese low fat	24
Cottage cheese dry	24
Figs dried	24
Figs fresh	24
Milk human	24
Avocados	24
Salmon raw	24
Swordfish	24
Anchovy in oil drained	25
Catfish	25
Eel fish	25
Haddock seafish	25
Pollock fish	25
Smelt fish	25
Snapper fish	25
Whitefish	25
Bass fish	25
Bluefish	25
Carp fish	25
Cod fish	25
Flat fish flounder & skin	26
Halibut flatfish	26
Herring fish	26
Mackerel fish	26
Perch fish	26
Pike fish	26
Sardines brine drained	26
Shark meat - flake	26
Tuna in spring water brine	26
Tomatoes red	26
Turnip root	26
Carob natural, e.g. powder or carob flour	26
Tomato juice	27
Bacon regular	27
Soy bean sprouts	27
Wild pheasant	27

Pork spare ribs	27
Cheese liver	27
Chicken dark meat	27
without skin	27
Chicken light meat	27
without skin	27
Chicken neck	27
Tomato paste	27
Summer sausage	27
Pineapple	28
Pork leg	28
Pork loin chop	28
Pork shoulder	28
Potatos	28
Chicken breasts	28
Cream of mushroom soup	28
Celery	28
Chicken drumstick	28
Turkey noodle soup	28
Beef flank steak	28
Beef noodle soup	28
Beef porterhouse steak	29
Beef rib roast	29
Beef short ribs	29
Beef sirloin steak	29
Beef sound steak	29
Beef soup with vegetable	29
Beef T-bone steak	29
Chicken gumbo sausages	29
Chicken noodle soup	29
Cream of asparagus soup	29
Knockwurst thick sausage	29
Potato baked	29
Beef chuck roast	30
Beef tenderloin	30
Chicken legs	30
Chicken light meat	30
Ham boneless	30
Persimmon fruit	30
Squash summer	30
Chicken canned boned	30

Chicken hearts	30
Cream of chicken soup	30
Turkey dark meat	30
Bratwurst cooked	30
Chicken thighs	31
Italian sausages cooked	31
Pork sausage	31
Turkey canned boned	31
Turkey light meat	31
Wild quail	31
Chicken dark meat	31
Beef & pork sausage	31
Goose farmed	31
Beef & pork bologna	31
Peaches dried	31
Beans with frankfurters	31
Black bean soup	32
Peaches fruit	32
Beef bologna	32
Beef corned brisket	32
Beef frankfurter	32
Beef ground lean	32
Beef ground regular	32
Chicken livers	32
Cream of celery soup	32
Duck's livers	32
Pastrami red meat	32
Goose livers	32
Mortadella pork sausage	33
Turkey liver	33
Plums fruit	33
Pork bratwurst	33
Beef dried	33
Beef smoked chopped	33
Chicken back	33
Green beans	33
Pork bacon	33
Polish sausage	33
Pork bologna	33
Salami dry	33
Scallops	34

shell-fish	34
Braunsch-weiger	34
Chicken wings	34
Duck farmed	34
Lentils sprouts	34
Lettuce romaine bitter	34
Caviar black & red	34
Lettuce common	34
Cauliflower	34
Vienna sausages	34
Guava fruit	34
Liver	35
New England clam chowder	35
Abalone shell-fish	35
Cream of potato soup	35
Spinach plant	35
Beef & pork frankfurter	35
Kale cabbage	35
Klobasa Slovak sausage smoked & spicy	35
Egg white	35
Eggs whole	35
Cabbage chinese	35
Corn	35
Eggs whole dried	36
Sweet potatoes	36
Watermelon red	36
Turnip greens	36
Oysters	36
Bananas	36
Chicken rice soup	36
Clams mollusc	36
Asparagus	36
Oats flakes	36
Beet greens	36
Endive salad plant	37
Leeks	37
Mayonnaise common	37
Pumpkins	37
Vegetarian veggie soup	37
Recipes with Lysine & Arginine Ratios	38

Breakfast Meals 38
    Greek Yogurt and Mango Breakfast Bowl 38
    Apricot and Cream Cheese Toast 38
    Apple Yogurt Parfait 38
    Eggs and Spinach Scramble 39
    Egg and Vegetable Omelette 39
    Spinach and Mushroom Omelette 39

Lunch Meals 41
    Cheese & Papaya Salad 41
    Cantaloupe and Greek Yogurt Smoothie 41
    Mozzarella and Pear Salad 41
    Chicken and Avocado Salad 42
    Shrimp and Quinoa Salad 42
    Tuna Salad 42
    Turkey and Avocado Sandwich 43
    Grilled Chicken Caesar Wrap 43

Dinner Meals 44
    Tofu and Broccoli Stir-Fry 44
    Greek Salad 44
    Chickpea Salad 44
    Quinoa and Black Bean Salad 45
    Mediterranean Chickpea Salad 45
    Roasted Chicken Breast with Steamed Broccoli 46
    Quinoa and Vegetable Stir-Fry 46
    Grilled Shrimp Skewers with Quinoa Salad 47
    Turkey Meatballs with Zucchini Noodles 47
    Grilled Portobello Mushrooms with Quinoa Salad 48
    Grilled Salmon with Lemon 48
    Beef Stir Fry with Bell Peppers 49
    Pork Chop with Roasted Sweet Potatoes 49
    Grilled Chicken Breast with Quinoa and Steamed Broccoli 50
    Salmon with Brown Rice and Roasted Asparagus 50
    Shrimp Stir Fry with Vegetables 51
    Grilled Lamb Chops with Couscous and Grilled Zucchini 51
    Tofu Stir-Fry with Brown Rice 51
    Baked Chicken Breast with Steamed Broccoli 52
    Salmon and Asparagus Foil Pack 52
    Greek Salad with Grilled Chicken 53
    Lentil and Vegetable Curry 53
    Stuffed Bell Peppers with Ground Turkey 54
    Turkey and Vegetable Skewers 54

    Lentil and Vegetable Curry   55
    Quinoa Stuffed Bell Peppers   56
    Turkey and Spinach Meatballs   56
    Salmon and Asparagus Foil Packets   57
    Vegetable Stir-Fry   57

Snacks   **59**
    Apple and Cottage Cheese Plate   59
    Pineapple and Ham Skewers   59

Soups   **59**
    Chicken and Vegetable Soup   59
    Lentil Soup   60

A word from Kayleigh Lee

As someone who actively suffers from the herpes virus, I am absolutely obsessed with using any and every method to heal my body.

Not long after my diagnosis I started learning about the virus and realised how much food triggered most of my outbreaks. I could literally eat green peas and get tingling sensations all over my body in a matter of hours!

I learned the hard way the importance of watching what you eat. However, this is not to say that all who carry this virus are triggered by food. With some, it can be stress, the sun, hormones, etc.

If you suspect food may be a trigger for you then this book is for you! It will give you some direction in knowing what may be triggering outbreaks, what foods to avoid and which ones to eat more of.

The Role of Amino Acids in Herpes Replication

Amino acids play a crucial role in the replication of viruses, including the herpes simplex virus (HSV). HSV requires certain amino acids, such as arginine, to replicate. Arginine is an essential amino acid that is involved in multiple cellular processes, including the synthesis of nitric oxide and polyamines. Nitric oxide is a molecule that helps relax blood vessels and improve blood flow, while polyamines are involved in cell growth and proliferation. Arginine is also involved in the synthesis of proteins, creatine, and urea, and is important for immune function and wound healing.

Lysine and arginine are two amino acids that are closely related and have a delicate balance in the body. Lysine has antiviral activity in vitro from antagonism of arginine metabolism. HSV replication requires the synthesis of arginine-rich proteins, and arginine is required for the virus to replicate. Lysine and arginine compete for absorption in the body, and increasing your intake of lysine can help reduce the amount of arginine available for the virus to use. This can help prevent the virus from replicating and reduce the frequency and severity of herpes outbreaks.

The Importance of Lysine and Arginine in Herpes Replication

The importance of lysine and arginine in herpes replication lies in their antagonistic relationship. Lysine has antiviral activity in vitro from antagonism of arginine metabolism. HSV replication requires the synthesis of arginine-rich proteins, and arginine is required for the virus to replicate. Lysine and arginine compete for absorption in the body, and increasing your intake of lysine can help reduce the amount of arginine available for the virus to use. This can help prevent the virus from replicating and reduce the frequency and severity of herpes outbreaks.

How Lysine Can Help Prevent Herpes Outbreaks

Lysine can help prevent herpes outbreaks by inhibiting the replication of the virus. Lysine supplementation can help reduce the frequency and severity of herpes outbreaks by reducing the availability of arginine for the virus to use. This can help prevent the virus from replicating and reduce the frequency and severity of herpes outbreaks. Lysine can also help boost the immune system, which can help prevent herpes outbreaks.

Scientific Evidence for Lysine and Herpes

Lysine has been recognized since 1952 as a potent inhibitor of viral replication. In 1958, researchers demonstrated that adding arginine to cultured HSV increased viral replication, while adding lysine decreased viral replication. Since then, numerous studies have been conducted to investigate the potential benefits of lysine for preventing and managing herpes outbreaks.

Some studies have shown that lysine supplementation can help reduce the frequency and severity of herpes outbreaks. However, other studies have found that lysine supplementation is ineffective for prophylaxis or treatment of herpes simplex lesions with doses of less than 1 g/d without low-arginine diets. Doses in excess of 3 g/d appear to improve patients' subjective experience of the disease.

The Effect of Lysine on Herpes Outbreaks

Lysine is an essential amino acid that is not produced by the body, so it must be obtained through diet or supplements. Lysine has gained popularity as a cheap and possibly effective agent in the treatment and prophylaxis of recurrent HSV. Lysine works by inhibiting the replication of the herpes simplex virus. HSV replication requires the synthesis of arginine-rich proteins, and arginine is required for the virus to replicate. Lysine and arginine compete for absorption in the body, and increasing your intake of lysine can help reduce the amount of arginine available for the virus to use. This can help prevent the virus from replicating and reduce the frequency and severity of herpes outbreaks.

The Significance of the Lysine/Arginine Ratio in Foods

The lysine/arginine ratio in foods is significant for individuals with herpes. Some people with herpes have found that avoiding foods high in the amino acid arginine may reduce recurrences. Higher levels of arginine are found in foods such as chocolate and many types of nuts. Excessive coffee (caffeine), red wine, and smoking are also triggers for some people. Lysine-rich foods include meat, fish, dairy products, and legumes. Maintaining a healthy diet that is rich in lysine and low in arginine can help prevent herpes outbreaks.

Tips for Maintaining a Lysine-Rich Diet

Maintaining a lysine-rich diet can help prevent herpes outbreaks. Lysine-rich foods include meat, fish, dairy products, and legumes. Some tips for maintaining a lysine-rich diet include:

- Eating lean meats, such as chicken and turkey
- Eating fish, such as salmon and tuna
- Consuming low-fat dairy products, such as milk, cheese, and yogurt
- Eating legumes, such as beans and lentils
- Avoiding foods high in arginine, such as chocolate and many types of nuts
- Consuming lysine supplements if necessary

Recommended Daily Intake of Lysine Through Supplementation

The recommended daily intake of lysine through supplementation varies depending on the individual's needs. Some studies have found that doses in excess of 3 g/d appear to improve patients' subjective experience of the disease. However, other studies have found that lysine supplementation is ineffective for prophylaxis or treatment of herpes simplex lesions with doses of less than 1 g/d without low-arginine diets. It is important to consult with a healthcare provider before taking lysine supplements to determine the appropriate dosage.

In conclusion, lysine works to prevent herpes outbreaks by inhibiting the replication of the herpes simplex virus. The lysine/arginine ratio in foods is significant for individuals with herpes, and maintaining a lysine-rich diet can help prevent herpes outbreaks. The recommended daily intake of lysine through supplementation varies depending on the individual's needs, and it is important to consult with a healthcare provider before taking lysine supplements to determine the appropriate dosage.

How to Use this Guide

This table provides information on the lysine (L-lysine) to arginine (L-arginine) ratios in various food items, along with their weight and the amount of lysine and arginine they contain. It is designed to help individuals who are trying to manage their intake of these two essential amino acids. This can be particularly useful for people dealing with conditions such as herpes, where some research suggests that a diet higher in lysine and lower in arginine might help control outbreaks.

The columns in the table are as follows:

Food Item: The type of food.

L-lysine vs. L-arginine in food product %-Ratio (Lys/Arg): This represents the ratio of lysine to arginine in the food item. A ratio above 1 means that the food has more lysine than arginine, while a ratio below 1 means the food has more arginine than lysine. The ratio is given as a percentage; for example, a ratio of 1 would be presented as 100%.

Item Weight (g & oz): The weight of the food item being considered, presented in both grams and ounces.

L-Lysine amount (mg & oz): The amount of lysine contained in the given weight of the food item, presented in both milligrams and ounces.

L-Arginine amount (mg & oz): The amount of arginine contained in the given weight of the food item, presented in both milligrams and ounces.

Here's how to read each row:

For example, in the case of "Abalone shell-fish", 100g (or 3.52oz) of this food contains 1282mg (or .0452oz) of lysine and 1247mg (or .0439oz) of arginine. The lysine to arginine ratio in this food product is 109% (or 1.09), indicating that it contains slightly more lysine than arginine.

In contrast, "Almonds nuts" contain considerably more arginine than lysine. 200g (or 7.05oz) of almonds contain 1332mg (or .0469oz) of lysine and a much larger 4986mg (or .1758oz) of arginine, giving a lysine to arginine ratio of just 27% (or 0.27).

Finally, "Anchovy in oil drained" has a lysine to arginine ratio of 154% (or 1.54), meaning it contains more lysine than arginine. In a 25g (or 0.88oz) serving, there are 664mg (or .0234oz) of lysine and 433mg (or .0152oz) of arginine.

When trying to increase lysine relative to arginine in your diet, you would aim to consume foods with a higher Lys/Arg ratio. It's important to remember that this is just one strategy, and any dietary changes should be part of a balanced and nutritious eating plan. As always, it's wise to consult with a healthcare professional or a dietitian before making significant dietary changes.

Foods with the Highest Lysine to Arginine Ratio

L-lysine vs. L-arginine in food product	%-Ratio Lys/Arg	Item Weight g & oz	L-Lysine amount mg & oz	L-Arginine amount mg & oz
Margarine	300% 3.00	10g 0.350oz	6mg .0002oz	2mg .0000oz
Yogurt fruit low fat	298% 2.98	100g 3.52oz	356mg .0125oz	119mg .0041oz
Yogurt plain	298% 2.98	100g 3.52oz	311mg .0109oz	104mg .0036oz
Yogurt plain skim	297% 2.97	100g 3.52oz	511mg .0180oz	172mg .0060oz
Yogurt plain low fat	295% 2.95	100g 3.52oz	467mg .0164oz	158mg .0055oz
Cheese swiss	279% 2.79	50g 1.76oz	1308mg .oz	469mg .oz
Cheese gruyere 6+ months aged	278% 2.78	50g 1.76oz	1372mg .0483oz	492mg .0173oz
Cheese American spread	276% 2.76	50g 1.76oz	763mg .0269oz	276mg .0097oz
Cheese edam	276% 2.76	50g 1.76oz	1346mg .0474oz	487mg .0171oz
Cheese gouda Dutch	276%	50g	1342mg	487mg

	2.76	1.76oz	.0473oz	.0171oz
Whey sweet dry	275%	50g	481mg	175mg
	2.75	1.76oz	.0169oz	.0061oz
Cheese blue	260%	50g	939mg	360mg
	2.60	1.76oz	.0331oz	.0126oz
Cheese provolone 2-3 months	259%	50g	480mg	185mg
	2.59	1.76oz	.0169oz	.0065oz
Papaya fruit called Pawpaw in Australia	253%	500g	83mg	33mg
	2.53	17.63oz	.0029oz	.0011oz
Cheese brie	252%	50g	938mg	371mg
	2.52	1.76oz	.0330oz	.0130oz
Cheese camermbert	252%	50g	894mg	355mg
	2.52	1.76oz	.0315oz	.0125oz
Cheese parmesan	251%	50g	1673mg	664mg
	2.51	1.76oz	.0590oz	.0234oz
Cheese parmesan grated	249%	10g	384mg	154mg
	2.49	0.35oz	.0135oz	.0054oz
Cheese goat brown	248%	50g	412mg	166mg
	2.48	1.76oz	.0145oz	.0058oz
Cheese brick	243%	50g	1075mg	442mg
	2.43	1.76oz	.0379oz	.0155oz
Milk goat's	243%	250g	725mg	298mg
	2.43	8.81oz	.0255oz	.0105oz

Cheese muenster orange with white	242% 2.42	50g 1.76oz	1082mg .0381oz	446mg .0157oz
Beets	240% 2.40	100g 3.52oz	53mg .0018oz	22mg .0007oz
Cheese limburger stinky-cheese	240% 2.40	50g 1.76oz	848mg .0299oz	354mg .0124oz
Cheese port du salut	240% 2.40	50g 1.76oz	1005mg .0354oz	419mg .0147oz
Cheese tilsit yellow semi-soft	240% 2.40	50g 1.76oz	1032mg .0364oz	430mg .0151oz
Cheese American processed	238% 2.38	50g 1.76oz	1112mg .0392oz	469mg .0165oz
Cheese swiss processed	238% 2.38	50g 1.76oz	1242mg .0438oz	523mg .0184oz
Cheese mozzarella	237% 2.37	50g 1.76oz	998mg .0352oz	421mg .0148oz
Cheese mozzarella grated	237% 2.37	50g 1.76oz	1248mg .0440oz	526mg .0185oz
Cream cheese	237% 2.37	50g 1.76oz	342mg .0120oz	144mg .0050oz
Cheese neufchatel soft white French	236% 2.36	50g 1.76oz	451mg .0159oz	191mg .0067oz

Butter common	225%	20g	13mg	6mg
	2.25	0.70oz	.0004oz	.0002oz
Cheese colby	221%	50g	1002mg	453mg
	2.21	1.76oz	.0353oz	.0159oz
Cheese monterey Jack semi-hard	221%	50g	1032mg	467mg
	2.21	1.76oz	.0364oz	.0164oz
Buttermilk	220%	200g	554mg	252mg
	2.20	7.05oz	.0195oz	.0088oz
Cheese cheddar	220%	50g	1050mg	476mg
	2.20	1.76oz	.0370oz	.0167oz
Cheese cheshire	220%	50g	983mg	446mg
	2.20	1.76oz	.0346oz	.0157oz
Half & half cream	220%	250g	586mg	267mg
	2.20	8.81oz	.0206oz	.0094oz
Milk skim	220%	250g	675mg	307mg
	2.20	8.81oz	.0238oz	.0108oz
Sherbet powder	220%	10g	9mg	4mg
	2.20	0.35oz	.0003oz	.0001oz
Ice cream	219%	200g	572mg	261mg
	2.19	7.05oz	.0201oz	.0092oz
Milk condensed	219%	250g	1569mg	715mg
	2.19	8.81oz	.0553oz	.0252oz
Milk dry instant non fat	219%	100g	2779mg	1270mg
	2.19	3.52oz	.0980oz	.0447oz

Milk dry non fat	219% 2.19	100g 3.52oz	2867mg .1011oz	1308mg .0461oz
Milk evaporated	219% 2.19	250g 8.81oz	1351mg .0476oz	617mg .0217oz
Milk evaporated skim	219% 2.19	250g 8.81oz	1490mg .0525oz	681mg .0240oz
Milk iced	219% 2.19	250g 8.81oz	780mg .0275oz	356mg .0125oz
Milk low fat	219% 2.19	250g 8.81oz	659mg .0232oz	301mg .0106oz
Milk whole	219% 2.19	250g 8.81oz	652mg .0229oz	298mg .0105oz
Milk whole dry	219% 2.19	100g 3.52oz	2085mg .0735oz	953mg .0336oz
Whipping cream heavy	219% 2.19	100g 3.52oz	387mg .0136oz	177mg .0062oz
Whipping cream light	219% 2.19	100g 3.52oz	171mg .0060oz	78mg .0027oz
Ice cream rich	218% 2.18	200g 7.05oz	442mg .0155oz	202mg .0071oz
Mango fruit	218% 2.18	500g 17.63oz	141mg .0049oz	65mg .0022oz
Whipped cream pressurized	217% 2.17	100g 3.52oz	253mg .0089oz	116mg .0040oz

Apricots fruit	215% 2.15	500g 17.63oz	451mg .0159oz	210mg .0074oz
Apples	213% 2.13	500g 17.63oz	57mg .0020.oz	27mg .0009oz
Coffee cream	213% 2.13	10g 0.35oz	21mg .0007oz	10mg .0003oz
Cheese ricotta	212% 2.12	50g 1.76oz	668mg .0235oz	315mg .0111oz
Cheese ricotta part skim	212% 2.12	50g 1.76oz	674mg .0237oz	319mg .0112oz
Milk chocolate flavour	209% 2.09	200g 7.05oz	503mg .0177oz	229mg .0080oz
Pears dried	207% 2.07	200g 7.05oz	132mg .0046oz	64mg .0022oz
Eggnog milk drink	202% 2.02	1/4 L 8.45 fl oz	746mg .0263oz	372mg .0131oz
Apple sauce unsweetened	200% 2.00	500g 17.63oz	49mg .0017oz	24mg .0008oz
Crabapple fruit slices	200% 2.00	100g 3.52oz	24mg .0008oz	12mg .0004oz
Loquat fruit	200% 2.00	50g 1.76oz	6mg .0002oz	3mg .0001oz
Apples dried	195% 1.95	500g 17.63oz	289mg .0101oz	148mg .0052oz

Pears fruit	192% 1.92	200g 7.05oz	25mg .0008oz	13mg .0004oz
Milk carob flavour	187% 1.87	1/4 L 8.45 fl oz	343mg .0120oz	182mg .0064oz
Apricots dried	182% 1.82	500g 17.63oz	1272mg .0448oz	700mg .0246oz
Cottage cheese creamed	178% 1.78	50g 1.76oz	504mg .0177oz	283mg .0099oz
Cottage cheese low fat	178% 1.78	50g 1.76oz	555mg .0195oz	312mg .0110oz
Cottage cheese dry	177% 1.77	50g 1.76oz	696mg .0245oz	393mg .0138oz
Figs dried	174% 1.74	50g 1.76oz	60mg .0021oz	34mg .0011oz
Figs fresh	173% 1.73	50g 1.76oz	14mg .0004oz	8mg .0002oz
Milk human	160% 1.60	250g 8.81oz	170mg .0059oz	107mg .0037oz
Avocados	159% 1.59	500g 17.63oz	347mg .0122oz	218mg .0076oz
Salmon raw	155% 1.55	100g 3.52oz	1823mg .0643oz	1176mg .0414oz
Swordfish	155% 1.55	100g 3.52oz	1823mg .0643oz	1176mg .0414oz

Anchovy in oil drained	154%	25g	664mg	433mg
	1.54	0.88oz	.0234oz	.0152oz
Catfish	154%	100g	1670mg	1088mg
	1.54	3.52oz	.0589oz	.0383oz
Eel fish	154%	100g	1694mg	1103mg
	1.54	3.52oz	.0597oz	.0389oz
Haddock seafish	154%	100g	1741mg	1130mg
	1.54	3.52oz	.0614oz	.0398oz
Pollock fish	154%	100g	1788mg	1163mg
	1.54	3.52oz	.0630oz	.0410oz
Smelt fish	154%	100g	1623mg	1055mg
	1.54	3.52oz	.0572oz	.0372oz
Snapper fish	154%	100g	1882mg	1223mg
	1.54	3.52oz	.0663oz	.0431oz
Whitefish	154%	100g	1752mg	1142mg
	1.54	3.52oz	.0617oz	.0402oz
Bass fish	153%	100g	1380mg	902mg
	1.53	3.52oz	.0486oz	.0318oz
Bluefish	153%	100g	1835mg	1200mg
	1.53	3.52oz	.0647oz	.0423oz
Carp fish	153%	100g	1635mg	1067mg
	1.53	3.52oz	.0576oz	.0376oz
Cod fish	153%	100g	1635mg	1065mg
	1.53	3.52oz	.0576oz	.0375oz

Flat fish flounder & skin	153%	100g	1729mg	1128mg
	1.53	3.52oz	.0609oz	.0397oz
Halibut flatfish	153%	100g	1905mg	1247mg
	1.53	3.52oz	.0671oz	.0439oz
Herring fish	153%	100g	1647mg	1075mg
	1.53	3.52oz	.0580oz	.0379oz
Mackerel fish	153%	100g	1705mg	1113mg
	1.53	3.52oz	.0601oz	.0392oz
Perch fish	153%	100g	1705mg	1115mg
	1.53	3.52oz	.0601oz	.0393oz
Pike fish	153%	100g	1764mg	1151mg
	1.53	3.52oz	.0622oz	.0406oz
Sardines brine drained	153%	50g	1129mg	737mg
	1.53	1.76oz	.0398oz	.0259oz
Shark meat - flake	153%	100g	1929mg	1258mg
	1.53	3.52oz	.0689oz	.0443oz
Tuna in spring water brine	153%	100g	2715mg	1769mg
	1.53	3.52oz	.0957oz	.0623oz
Tomatoes red	152%	100g	33mg	21mg
	1.52	3.52oz	.0011oz	.0007oz
Turnip root	152%	200g	72mg	47mg
	1.52	7.05oz	.0025oz	.0016oz
Carob natural, e.g. powder or carob flour	151%	100g	1960mg	1300mg
	1.51	3.52oz	.0691oz	.0459oz

Tomato juice	150% 1.50	1/4 Liter 8.45 fl oz	55mg .0019oz	37mg .0013oz
Bacon regular	145% 1.45	500g 17.63oz	8116mg .2862oz	5616mg .1980oz
Soy bean sprouts	145% 1.45	100g 3.52oz	551mg .0194oz	380mg .0134oz
Wild pheasant	143% 1.43	100g 3.52oz	2013mg .0710oz	1412mg .0498oz
Pork spare ribs	142% 1.42	500g 17.63oz	5736mg .2023oz	4050mg .1428oz
Cheese liver	141% 1.41	50g 1.76oz	596mg .0210oz	423mg .0149oz
Chicken dark meat without skin	141% 1.41	200g 7.05oz	3412mg .1203oz	2422 .0854oz
Chicken light meat without skin	141% 1.41	100g 3.52oz	1965mg .0693oz	1397mg .0492oz
Chicken neck	141% 1.41	100g 3.52oz	377mg .0132oz	268mg .0094oz
Tomato paste	141% 1.41	100g 3.52oz	107mg .0037oz	76mg .0026oz
Summer sausage	140% 1.40	100g 3.52oz	1382mg .0487oz	991mg .0349oz

Pineapple	139% 1.39	200g 7.05oz	50mg .0017oz	36mg .0012oz
Pork leg	137% 1.37	500g 17.63oz	8315mg .2933oz	6090mg .2148oz
Pork loin chop	136% 1.36	500g 17.63oz	6457mg .2277oz	4735mg .1670oz
Pork shoulder	136% 1.36	500g 17.63oz	7863mg .2773oz	5770mg .2035oz
Potatos	136% 1.36	200g 7.05oz	253mg .0089oz	186mg .0065oz
Chicken breasts	134% 1.34	200g 7.05oz	2762mg .0974oz	2066mg .0728oz
Cream of mushroom soup	134% 1.34	200g 7.05oz	104mg .0036oz	77mg .0027oz
Celery	133% 1.33	100g 3.52oz	26mg .0009oz	20mg .0007oz
Chicken drumstick	133% 1.33	200g 7.05oz	2109mg .0743oz	1585mg .0559oz
Turkey noodle soup	133% 1.33	100g 3.52oz	86mg .0030oz	65mg .0022oz
Beef flank steak	132% 1.32	500g 17.63oz	8006mg .2824oz	6057mg .2136oz
Beef noodle soup	132% 1.32	200g 7.05oz	214mg .0075oz	155mg .0054oz

Beef porterhouse steak	132% 1.32	500g 17.63oz	7224mg .2548oz	5484mg .1934oz
Beef rib roast	132% 1.32	500g 17.63oz	6659mg .2348oz	5065mg .1786oz
Beef short ribs	132% 1.32	500g 17.63oz	5980mg .2109oz	4548mg .1604oz
Beef sirloin steak	132% 1.32	500g 17.63oz	7577mg .2672oz	5759mg .2031oz
Beef sound steak	132% 1.32	500g 17.63oz	8061mg .2843oz	6112mg .2155oz
Beef soup with vegetable	132% 1.32	200g 7.05oz	282mg .0099oz	214mg .0075oz
Beef T-bone steak	132% 1.32	500g 17.63oz	6971mg .2458oz	5297mg .1868oz
Chicken gumbo sausages	132% 1.32	200g 7.05oz	132mg .0046oz	100mg .0035oz
Chicken noodle soup	132% 1.32	200g 7.05oz	181mg .0063oz	137mg .0048oz
Cream of asparagus soup	132% 1.32	100g 3.52oz	46mg .0016oz	34mg .0011oz
Knockwurst thick sausage	132% 1.32	200g 7.05oz	1864mg .0657oz	1417mg .0499oz
Potato baked	132% 1.32	200g 7.05oz	280mg .0098oz	211mg .0074oz

Beef chuck roast	131% 1.31	500g 17.63oz	7599mg .2680oz	5781mg .2039oz
Beef tenderloin	131% 1.31	500g 17.63oz	7698mg .2715oz	5859mg .2066oz
Chicken legs	131% 1.31	200g 7.05oz	2138mg .0754oz	1636mg .0577oz
Chicken light meat	131% 1.31	100g 3.52oz	1655mg .0583oz	1267mg .0446oz
Ham boneless	131% 1.31	500g 17.63oz	7433mg .2621oz	5693mg .2008oz
Persimmon fruit	131% 1.31	200g 7.05oz	55mg .0019oz	42mg .0014oz
Squash summer	131% 1.31	50g 1.76oz	32mg .0011oz	25mg .0008oz
Chicken canned boned	130% 1.30	200g 7.05oz	3521mg .1241oz	2704mg .0953oz
Chicken hearts	130% 1.30	10g 0.35oz	131mg .0046oz	101mg .0035oz
Cream of chicken soup	130% 1.30	100g 3.52oz	88mg .0031oz	68mg .0023oz
Turkey dark meat	130% 1.30	100g 3.52oz	1723mg .0607oz	1329mg .0468oz
Bratwurst cooked	129% 1.29	100g 3.52oz	1070mg .0377oz	830mg .0292oz

Chicken thighs	129%	100g	1091mg	850mg
	1.29	3.52oz	.0384oz	.0299oz
Italian sausages cooked	129%	100g	1522mg	1182mg
	1.29	3.52oz	.0536oz	.0416oz
Pork sausage	129%	500g	4502mg	3500mg
	1.29	17.63oz	.1588oz	.1234oz
Turkey canned boned	129%	100g	2140mg	1662mg
	1.29	3.52oz	.0754oz	.0586oz
Turkey light meat	129%	100g	1967mg	1522mg
	1.29	3.52oz	.0693oz	.0536oz
Wild quail	129%	200g	3288mg	2558mg
	1.29	7.05oz	.1159oz	.0902oz
Chicken dark meat	128%	200g	2687mg	2100mg
	1.28	7.05oz	.0947oz	.0740oz
Beef & pork sausage	127%	100g	1084mg	853mg
	1.27	3.52oz	.0382oz	.0300oz
Goose farmed	127%	500g	6265mg	4921mg
	1.27	oz	.2209oz	.1735oz
Beef & pork bologna	126%	200g	1785mg	1414mg
	1.26	7.05oz	.0629oz	.0498oz
Peaches dried	126%	100g	116mg	92mg
	1.26	3.52oz	.0040oz	.0032oz
Beans with frankfurters	125%	250g	415mg	331mg
	1.25	8.81oz	.0146oz	.0116oz

Black bean soup	125%	200g	336mg	268mg
	1.25	7.05oz	.0118oz	.0094oz
Peaches fruit	125%	100g	17mg	13mg
	1.25	3.52oz	.0005oz	.0004oz
Beef bologna	124%	500g	4535mg	3660mg
	1.24	17.63oz	.1599oz	.1291oz
Beef corned brisket	124%	500g	5616mg	4515mg
	1.24	17.63oz	.1980oz	.1592oz
Beef frankfurter	124%	200g	1728mg	1395mg
	1.24	7.05oz	.0609oz	.0492oz
Beef ground lean	124%	200g	2955mg	2389mg
	1.24	7.05oz	.1042oz	.0842oz
Beef ground regular	124%	200g	2761mg	2230mg
	1.24	7.05oz	.0973oz	.0786oz
Chicken livers	124%	100g	1283mg	1040mg
	1.24	3.52oz	.0452oz	.0366oz
Cream of celery soup	124%	100g	30mg	24mg
	1.24	3.52oz	.0010oz	.0008oz
Duck's livers	124%	50g	709mg	573mg
	1.24	1.76oz	.0250oz	.0202oz
Pastrami red meat	124%	50g	669mg	539mg
	1.24	1.76oz	.0235oz	.0190oz
Goose livers	123%	100g	1233mg	1002mg
	1.23	3.52oz	.0434oz	.0353oz

Mortadella pork sausage	123% 1.23	30g 1.05oz	383mg .0135oz	311mg .0109oz
Turkey liver	123% 1.23	100g 3.52oz	1510mg .0532oz	1225mg .0432oz
Plums fruit	122% 1.22	200g 7.05oz	3000mg .1058oz	2467mg .0870oz
Pork bratwurst	121% 11.21	100g 3.52oz	1153mg .0406oz	957mg .0337oz
Beef dried	121% 1.21	200g 7.05oz	4807mg .1695oz	3978mg .1403oz
Beef smoked chopped	121% 1.21	200g 7.05oz	3335mg .1176oz	2757mg .0972oz
Chicken back	121% 1.21	200g 7.05oz	1231mg .0434oz	1016mg .0358oz
Green beans	121% 1.21	100g 3.52oz	88mg .0031oz	72mg .0025oz
Pork bacon	121% 1.21	500g 17.63oz	3193mg .1126oz	2643mg .0932oz
Polish sausage	120% 1.20	100g 3.52oz	1125mg .0396oz	935mg .0329oz
Pork bologna	120% 1.20	50g 1.76oz	608mg .0214oz	509mg .0179oz
Salami dry	120% 1.20	100g 3.52oz	1820mg .0641oz	1520mg .0536oz

Scallops shell-fish	120% 1.20	100g 3.52oz	1247mg .0439oz	1223mg .0431oz
Braunsch - weiger	119% 1.19	50g 1.76oz	460mg .0162oz	387mg .0136oz
Chicken wings	119% 1.19	100g 3.52oz	775mg .0273oz	650mg .0229oz
Duck farmed	118% 1.18	500g 17.63oz	4547mg .1603oz	3850mg .1358oz
Lentils sprouts	117% 1.17	100g 3.52oz	711mg .0250oz	610mg .0215oz
Lettuce romaine bitter	116% 1.16	200g 7.05oz	207mg .0073oz	178mg .0062oz
Caviar black & red	115% 1.15	10g 0.35oz	183mg .0064oz	157mg .0055oz
Lettuce common	115% 1.15	200g 7.05oz	160mg .0056oz	138mg .0048oz
Cauliflower	113% 1.13	100g 3.52oz	108mg .0038oz	96mg .0033oz
Vienna sausages	112% 1.12	100g 3.52oz	793mg .0279oz	706mg .0249oz
Guava fruit	111% 1.11	100g 3.52oz	18mg .0006oz	16mg .0005oz

Liver	111%	100g	1389mg	1256mg
	1.11	3.52oz	.0489oz	.0443oz
New England clam chowder	110%	200g	205mg	187mg
	1.10	7.05oz	.0072oz	.0065oz
Abalone shell-fish	109%	100g	1282mg	1247mg
	1.09	3.52oz	.0452oz	.0439oz
Cream of potato soup	109%	200g	83mg	76mg
	1.09	7.05oz	.0029oz	.0026oz
Spinach plant	109%	100g	178mg	163mg
	1.09	3.52oz	.0062oz	.0057oz
Beef & pork frankfurter	107%	100g	904mg	849mg
	1.07	3.52oz	.0318oz	.0299oz
Kale cabbage	107%	100g	197mg	183mg
	1.07	3.52oz	.0069oz	.0064oz
Klobasa Slovak sausage smoked & spicy	107%	200g	2042mg	1907mg
	1.07	7.05oz	.0720oz	.0672oz
Egg white	106%	20g	124mg	118mg
	1.06	0.70oz	.0043oz	.0041oz
Eggs whole	106%	45g	369mg	349mg
	1.06	1.58oz	.0130oz	.0123oz
Cabbage chinese	105%	100g	88mg	84mg
	1.05	3.52oz	.0031oz	.0029oz
Corn	105%	100g	136mg	129mg

		1.05	3.52oz	.0047oz	.0045oz
Eggs whole dried		105%	10g	310mg	294mg
		1.05	0.35oz	.0109oz	.0103oz
Sweet potatoes		105%	100g	80mg	77mg
		1.05	3.52oz	.0028oz	.0027oz
Watermelon red		105%	200g	123mg	117mg
		1.05	7.05oz	.0043oz	.0041oz
Turnip greens		104%	100g	98mg	94mg
		1.04	3.52oz	.0034oz	.0033oz
Oysters		103%	100g	528mg	515mg
		1.03	3.52oz	.0186oz	.0181oz
Bananas		102%	500g	157mg	154mg
		1.02	17.63oz	.0055oz	.0054oz
Chicken rice soup		102%	200g	208mg	195mg
		1.02	7.05oz	.0073oz	.0068oz
Clams mollusc		102%	200g	1911mg	1867mg
		1.02	7.05oz	.0674oz	.0658oz
Asparagus		101%	200g	289mg	286mg
		1.01	7.05oz	.0101oz	.0100oz
Oats flakes		101%	100g	1214mg	1206mg
		1.01	3.52oz	.0428oz	.0425oz
Beet greens		100%	100g	52mg	52mg
		1.00	3.52oz	.0018oz	.0018oz

Endive salad plant	100%	100g	63mg	63mg
	1.00	3.52oz	.0022oz	.0022oz
Leeks	100%	100g	78mg	78mg
	1.00	3.52oz	.0027oz	.0027oz
Mayonnaise common	100%	185g	1400mg	1400mg
	1.00	6.52oz	.0493oz	.0493oz
Pumpkins	100%	200g	78mg	78mg
	1.00	7.05oz	.0027oz	.0027oz
Vegetarian veggie soup	100%	100g	41mg	41mg
	1.00	3.52oz	.0014oz	.0014oz

Recipes with Lysine & Arginine Ratios

Breakfast Meals

Greek Yogurt and Mango Breakfast Bowl

Ingredients:

1 cup plain low-fat yogurt (467mg Lysine, 158mg Arginine), 1 medium-sized mango (282mg Lysine, 130mg Arginine)

Instructions:

- Peel and slice the mango.
- In a bowl, add the yogurt and top with the sliced mango. Serve immediately.

Lysine/Arginine: 749mg/288mg

Apricot and Cream Cheese Toast

Ingredients:

2 slices of gluten-free + nut-free bread, 2 tablespoons of cream cheese (171mg Lysine, 72mg Arginine), 4 fresh apricots (180mg Lysine, 84mg Arginine)

Instructions:

- Toast the slices of bread.
- Spread cream cheese on each toasted slice.
- Slice apricots and place on top of the cream cheese. Serve immediately.

Lysine/Arginine: 351mg/156mg

Apple Yogurt Parfait

Ingredients:

2 medium-sized apples (114mg Lysine, 54mg Arginine), 1 cup of plain low-fat yogurt (467mg Lysine, 158mg Arginine), 1 teaspoon of honey.

Instructions:

- Wash and slice the apples.

- In a glass, layer yogurt, sliced apples, and a drizzle of honey.
- Repeat the layers until you run out of ingredients, ending with a layer of yogurt and a drizzle of honey on top. Serve chilled.

Lysine/Arginine: 581mg/212mg

Eggs and Spinach Scramble

Ingredients:

2 large eggs (1234mg Lysine, 645mg Arginine), 1 cup spinach, 1 tablespoon olive oil, a pinch of salt and black pepper.

Instructions:

- Heat the oil in a pan over medium heat.
- Add the spinach and cook until wilted.
- Beat the eggs and pour them over the spinach. Stir until the eggs are cooked. Season with salt and pepper. Serve immediately.

Lysine/Arginine: 1234mg/645mg

Egg and Vegetable Omelette

Ingredients:

2 large eggs (1140mg Lysine, 704mg Arginine), 1/2 cup chopped mixed vegetables (e.g., bell peppers, onions, mushrooms) (40mg Lysine, 60mg Arginine), 1 tablespoon olive oil.

Instructions:

- Heat the olive oil in a non-stick skillet over medium heat.
- Add the chopped vegetables and sauté until they're tender.
- In a separate bowl, beat the eggs until well combined.
- Pour the beaten eggs into the skillet with the vegetables.
- Cook the omelette, lifting the edges and tilting the skillet to allow the uncooked eggs to flow to the edges.
- Once the eggs are set, fold the omelette in half and cook for another minute.
- Transfer the omelette to a plate and serve hot.

Lysine/Arginine: 1180mg/764mg

Spinach and Mushroom Omelette

Ingredients:

2 eggs (252mg Lysine, 170mg Arginine), 1 cup fresh spinach leaves (30mg Lysine, 20mg Arginine), 1/2 cup sliced mushrooms (20mg Lysine, 20mg Arginine), 1/4 cup shredded mozzarella cheese (140mg Lysine, 105mg Arginine), salt and pepper to taste, olive oil (for cooking).

Instructions:

- In a small bowl, whisk the eggs until well beaten. Season with salt and pepper.
- Heat olive oil in a non-stick skillet over medium heat.
- Add the sliced mushrooms to the skillet and cook until softened, about 2 minutes.
- Add the fresh spinach leaves to the skillet and cook until wilted, about 1 minute.
- Pour the beaten eggs over the mushrooms and spinach in the skillet.
- Sprinkle the shredded mozzarella cheese evenly over the eggs.
- Cook until the omelette is set and the cheese is melted, about 2-3 minutes.
- Carefully fold the omelette in half and transfer to a plate.
- Serve the spinach and mushroom omelette hot for a protein-rich breakfast or brunch.

Lysine/Arginine: 442mg/315mg

Lunch Meals

Cheese & Papaya Salad

Ingredients:

100g Gouda cheese (2684mg Lysine, 974mg Arginine), 1 medium-sized papaya (166mg Lysine, 66mg Arginine), 1 tablespoon olive oil, a pinch of salt and black pepper.

Instructions:

- Peel and slice the papaya.
- Slice the Gouda cheese.
- In a bowl, add the sliced cheese and papaya.
- Drizzle olive oil, sprinkle a pinch of salt and black pepper, and toss gently to combine. Serve immediately.

Lysine/Arginine: 2850mg/1040mg

Cantaloupe and Greek Yogurt Smoothie

Ingredients:

1 cup diced cantaloupe (123mg Lysine, 72mg Arginine), 1 cup plain low-fat Greek yogurt (1103mg Lysine, 473mg Arginine)

Instructions:

- In a blender, combine the cantaloupe and yogurt.
- Blend until smooth. Pour into a glass and serve immediately.

Lysine/Arginine: 1226mg/545mg

Mozzarella and Pear Salad

Ingredients:

100g mozzarella cheese (1996mg Lysine, 842mg Arginine), 2 medium-sized pears (50mg Lysine, 22mg Arginine), a handful of spinach, 1 tablespoon olive oil, a pinch of salt and black pepper.

Instructions:

- Slice the mozzarella cheese and pears.
- In a bowl, add spinach, sliced cheese, and pears.

- Drizzle olive oil, sprinkle a pinch of salt and black pepper, and toss gently to combine. Serve immediately.

Lysine/Arginine: 2046mg/864mg

Chicken and Avocado Salad

Ingredients:

100g chicken breast (2793mg Lysine, 1519mg Arginine), 1 small avocado (368mg Lysine, 160mg Arginine), a handful of spinach, 1 tablespoon olive oil, a pinch of salt and black pepper.

Instructions:

- Cook the chicken breast as per your liking and let it cool. Then, slice it.
- Slice the avocado.
- In a bowl, add spinach, sliced chicken, and avocado.
- Drizzle olive oil, sprinkle a pinch of salt and black pepper, and toss gently to combine. Serve immediately.

Lysine/Arginine: 3161mg/1679mg

Shrimp and Quinoa Salad

Ingredients:

100g shrimp (1693mg Lysine, 1710mg Arginine), 1/2 cup cooked quinoa (658mg Lysine, 451mg Arginine), 1 cup spinach, 1 tablespoon olive oil, a pinch of salt and black pepper.

Instructions:

- Cook the shrimp as per your liking.
- In a bowl, add spinach, cooked shrimp, and quinoa.
- Drizzle olive oil, sprinkle a pinch of salt and black pepper, and toss gently to combine. Serve immediately.

Lysine/Arginine: 2351mg/2161mg

Tuna Salad

Ingredients:

1 can of tuna in water (2725mg Lysine, 1910mg Arginine), 2 cups of mixed greens (80mg Lysine, 100mg Arginine), 1 tablespoon of olive oil, a pinch of salt and black pepper.

Instructions:

- Drain the tuna and place it in a bowl.
- Add the mixed greens, olive oil, salt, and pepper.
- Toss gently to combine and serve.

Lysine/Arginine: 2805mg/2010mg

Turkey and Avocado Sandwich

Ingredients:

2 slices of whole grain bread (150mg Lysine, 150mg Arginine), 100g turkey breast (2450mg Lysine, 1500mg Arginine), 1/2 avocado (200mg Lysine, 150mg Arginine).

Instructions:

- Toast the bread to your liking.
- Layer turkey breast and sliced avocado on one slice of bread.
- Top with the other slice. Cut in half if desired and serve.

Lysine/Arginine: 2800mg/1800mg

Grilled Chicken Caesar Wrap

Ingredients:

Grilled chicken breast (100g): Lysine - 2,150mg, Arginine - 2,070mg, Romaine lettuce, Caesar dressing and Whole wheat wrap

Instructions:

- Slice the grilled chicken breast into strips.
- Fill the whole wheat wrap with chicken, romaine lettuce, and drizzle with Caesar dressing.
- Roll it up tightly.

Lysine/Arginine: 2,150mg/2,070mg

Dinner Meals

Tofu and Broccoli Stir-Fry

Ingredients:

100g tofu (615mg Lysine, 340mg Arginine), 1 cup chopped broccoli (335mg Lysine, 230mg Arginine), 1 tablespoon soy sauce, 1 tablespoon vegetable oil.

Instructions:

- Heat the oil in a pan over medium heat.
- Add the tofu and stir-fry until it's lightly browned. Remove it from the pan and set it aside.
- In the same pan, add the broccoli and stir-fry for about 5 minutes until it's tender.
- Add the tofu back to the pan, add the soy sauce, and stir to combine. Serve immediately.

Lysine/Arginine: 950mg/570mg

Greek Salad

Ingredients:

2 cups mixed salad greens (20mg Lysine, 40mg Arginine), 1/4 cup diced cucumber (10mg Lysine, 10mg Arginine), 1/4 cup diced tomatoes (10mg Lysine, 20mg Arginine), 1/4 cup sliced red onion (10mg Lysine, 10mg Arginine), 1/4 cup crumbled feta cheese (150mg Lysine, 140mg Arginine), 2 tablespoons Kalamata olives (20mg Lysine, 20mg Arginine), 1 tablespoon extra virgin olive oil, 1 tablespoon lemon juice, salt, and pepper.

Instructions:

- In a large bowl, combine the mixed salad greens, diced cucumber, diced tomatoes, sliced red onion, crumbled feta cheese, and Kalamata olives.
- Drizzle the extra virgin olive oil and lemon juice over the salad.
- Season with salt and pepper to taste.
- Toss everything together until well coated.
- Serve the Greek salad chilled as a refreshing side dish or light meal.

Lysine/Arginine: 220mg/240mg

Chickpea Salad

Ingredients:

1 can chickpeas, drained and rinsed (1450mg Lysine, 440mg Arginine), 1 cucumber, diced (10mg Lysine, 20mg Arginine), 1 red bell pepper, diced (20mg Lysine, 30mg Arginine), 1/4 cup chopped red onion (10mg Lysine, 10mg Arginine), 1/4 cup chopped fresh parsley, 2 tablespoons lemon juice, 2 tablespoons olive oil, salt, and pepper.

Instructions:

- In a large bowl, combine the chickpeas, diced cucumber, diced red bell pepper, chopped red onion, and chopped fresh parsley.
- In a separate small bowl, whisk together the lemon juice, olive oil, salt, and pepper to make the dressing.
- Pour the dressing over the chickpea mixture and toss until well combined.
- Adjust the seasoning if needed.
- Serve the chickpea salad chilled as a refreshing and protein-packed dish.

Lysine/Arginine: 1490mg/500mg

Quinoa and Black Bean Salad

Ingredients:

1 cup cooked quinoa (1115mg Lysine, 685mg Arginine), 1 cup black beans, rinsed and drained (1155mg Lysine, 985mg Arginine), 1 bell pepper, diced (10mg Lysine, 20mg Arginine), 1 cucumber, diced (20mg Lysine, 10mg Arginine), 1/4 cup red onion, finely chopped (10mg Lysine, 10mg Arginine), 1/4 cup fresh cilantro, chopped, juice of 1 lime, 2 tablespoons olive oil, salt and pepper to taste.

Instructions:

- In a large bowl, combine the cooked quinoa, black beans, diced bell pepper, diced cucumber, chopped red onion, and chopped cilantro.
- In a small bowl, whisk together the lime juice, olive oil, salt, and pepper.
- Pour the dressing over the quinoa and black bean mixture and toss to combine.
- Adjust the seasoning to taste.
- Serve the quinoa and black bean salad as a refreshing and protein-packed dish.

Lysine/Arginine: 1310mg/1720mg

Mediterranean Chickpea Salad

Ingredients:

1 cup cooked chickpeas (1500mg Lysine, 950mg Arginine), 1/2 cup diced cucumbers (20mg Lysine, 20mg Arginine), 1/2 cup diced tomatoes (20mg Lysine, 40mg Arginine), 1/4 cup diced red onion (10mg Lysine, 10mg Arginine), 1/4 cup chopped Kalamata olives (20mg Lysine, 20mg Arginine), 2 tablespoons chopped fresh parsley, 2 tablespoons lemon juice, 2 tablespoons olive oil, salt, and pepper.

Instructions:

- In a large bowl, combine the cooked chickpeas, diced cucumbers, diced tomatoes, diced red onion, and chopped Kalamata olives.
- Add the chopped parsley and toss everything together.
- Drizzle the lemon juice and olive oil over the salad.
- Season with salt and pepper to taste.
- Mix well to combine all the flavors.
- Let the salad marinate in the refrigerator for at least 30 minutes before serving.

Lysine/Arginine: 1570mg/1040mg

Roasted Chicken Breast with Steamed Broccoli

Ingredients:

1 boneless, skinless chicken breast (2610mg Lysine, 2520mg Arginine), 1 cup broccoli florets (30mg Lysine, 30mg Arginine), olive oil, salt, and pepper.

Instructions:

- Preheat the oven to 425°F (220°C).
- Place the chicken breast on a baking sheet and drizzle with olive oil. Season with salt and pepper.
- Roast the chicken breast in the preheated oven for 20-25 minutes until cooked through and juices run clear.
- While the chicken is roasting, steam the broccoli florets until tender-crisp, about 5-7 minutes.
- Once the chicken is cooked, remove it from the oven and let it rest for a few minutes before slicing.
- Serve the roasted chicken breast with steamed broccoli for a protein-packed and nutritious meal.

Lysine/Arginine: 2640mg/2550mg

Quinoa and Vegetable Stir-Fry

Ingredients:

1 cup cooked quinoa (550mg Lysine, 550mg Arginine), 1 cup mixed vegetables (e.g., broccoli, bell peppers, carrots) (40mg Lysine, 60mg Arginine), 2 tablespoons soy sauce (170mg Lysine, 170mg Arginine), 1 tablespoon sesame oil, 1/2 teaspoon minced garlic, 1/2 teaspoon grated ginger, salt, and pepper.

Instructions:

- Heat sesame oil in a large skillet or wok over medium heat.
- Add the minced garlic and grated ginger to the skillet and sauté for 1 minute until fragrant.
- Add the mixed vegetables to the skillet and stir-fry for 5-7 minutes until they're crisp-tender.
- Stir in the cooked quinoa and soy sauce.
- Season with salt and pepper to taste.
- Cook for an additional 2-3 minutes, stirring continuously to combine all the flavors.
- Remove from heat and serve the quinoa and vegetable stir-fry hot.

Lysine/Arginine: 760mg/780mg

Grilled Shrimp Skewers with Quinoa Salad

Ingredients:

100g shrimp (2150mg Lysine, 1280mg Arginine), 1/2 cup cooked quinoa (550mg Lysine, 550mg Arginine), 1 cup mixed vegetables (e.g., cucumber, cherry tomatoes, red onion) (40mg Lysine, 60mg Arginine), 1 tablespoon lemon juice, 1 tablespoon olive oil.

Instructions:

- Preheat the grill to medium-high heat.
- Thread the shrimp onto skewers and brush them with olive oil.
- Grill the shrimp skewers for 2-3 minutes per side until they're pink and cooked through.
- In a bowl, combine the cooked quinoa, mixed vegetables, lemon juice, and olive oil. Toss well to coat.
- Serve the grilled shrimp skewers on a bed of quinoa salad.

Lysine/Arginine: 2740mg/1890mg

Turkey Meatballs with Zucchini Noodles

Ingredients:

150g ground turkey (3465mg Lysine, 2385mg Arginine), 1 medium zucchini (60mg Lysine, 80mg Arginine), 1/4 cup marinara sauce (optional), 1 tablespoon olive oil, fresh basil leaves for garnish.

Instructions:

- In a mixing bowl, combine the ground turkey with your choice of herbs, spices, and salt.
- Shape the turkey mixture into small meatballs.
- Heat olive oil in a skillet over medium heat.
- Add the turkey meatballs to the skillet and cook for 8-10 minutes, turning occasionally until they're cooked through.
- While the meatballs are cooking, use a spiralizer or vegetable peeler to create zucchini noodles.
- Heat a separate skillet over medium heat and sauté the zucchini noodles for 2-3 minutes until they're tender.
- Serve the turkey meatballs over zucchini noodles, and optionally, top with marinara sauce and fresh basil leaves.

Lysine/Arginine: 3525mg/2465mg

Grilled Portobello Mushrooms with Quinoa Salad

Ingredients:

2 large Portobello mushrooms (1580mg Lysine, 1390mg Arginine), 1/2 cup cooked quinoa (550mg Lysine, 550mg Arginine), 1 cup mixed vegetables (e.g., bell peppers, cherry tomatoes, red onion) (40mg Lysine, 60mg Arginine), 1 tablespoon balsamic vinegar, 1 tablespoon olive oil, fresh parsley for garnish.

Instructions:

- Preheat the grill to medium heat.
- Brush the Portobello mushrooms with olive oil and balsamic vinegar.
- Grill the mushrooms for 4-5 minutes per side until they're tender and juicy.
- In a bowl, combine the cooked quinoa, mixed vegetables, balsamic vinegar, and olive oil. Mix well to combine.
- Serve the grilled Portobello mushrooms over a bed of quinoa salad. Garnish with fresh parsley.

Lysine/Arginine: 2130mg/2000mg

Grilled Salmon with Lemon

Ingredients:

100g salmon (2140mg Lysine, 1473mg Arginine), 1/2 lemon, salt and pepper to taste.

Instructions:

- Preheat your grill to medium heat.
- Season the salmon with salt and pepper and squeeze the lemon juice over it.
- Grill the salmon for about 4-6 minutes per side, or until it's cooked to your liking. Serve immediately.

Lysine/Arginine: 2140mg/1473mg

Beef Stir Fry with Bell Peppers

Ingredients:

100g beef (2300mg Lysine, 1411mg Arginine), 1 bell pepper (30mg Lysine, 40mg Arginine), 1 tablespoon of soy sauce, 1 tablespoon of vegetable oil.

Instructions:

- Cut the beef into thin slices and season with salt and pepper.
- Heat the oil in a pan over medium heat.
- Add the beef and stir fry until it's cooked to your liking.
- Add the sliced bell pepper and stir fry for a couple more minutes until the peppers are tender.
- Add the soy sauce, stir well and serve immediately.

Lysine/Arginine: 2330mg/1451mg

Pork Chop with Roasted Sweet Potatoes

Ingredients:

100g pork chop (2770mg Lysine, 1751mg Arginine), 1 medium-sized sweet potato (80mg Lysine, 50mg Arginine).

Instructions:

- Preheat your oven to 200 degrees Celsius.
- Season the pork chop with salt and pepper and pan fry it until it's cooked to your liking.
- At the same time, roast the sweet potato in the oven until it's tender (about 30-40 minutes).

- Serve the pork chop with the roasted sweet potato.

Lysine/Arginine: 2850mg/1801mg

Grilled Chicken Breast with Quinoa and Steamed Broccoli

Ingredients:

1 chicken breast (3250mg Lysine, 2075mg Arginine), 1/2 cup cooked quinoa (550mg Lysine, 550mg Arginine), 1 cup steamed broccoli (100mg Lysine, 100mg Arginine).

Instructions:

- Preheat the grill to medium-high heat.
- Season the chicken breast with your choice of herbs and spices.
- Grill the chicken breast for about 6-8 minutes per side until it reaches an internal temperature of 165°F (74°C).
- Meanwhile, cook the quinoa according to package instructions.
- Steam the broccoli until it's tender yet still crisp.
- Slice the grilled chicken breast and serve it with cooked quinoa and steamed broccoli.

Lysine/Arginine: 3900mg/2725mg

Salmon with Brown Rice and Roasted Asparagus

Ingredients:

100g salmon fillet (2325mg Lysine, 1445mg Arginine), 1/2 cup cooked brown rice (150mg Lysine, 150mg Arginine), 1 cup roasted asparagus (120mg Lysine, 160mg Arginine).

Instructions:

- Preheat the oven to 200 degrees Celsius.
- Place the salmon fillet on a baking sheet lined with parchment paper.
- Season the salmon with salt, pepper, and your choice of herbs or spices.
- Bake the salmon for 12-15 minutes until it flakes easily with a fork.
- While the salmon is baking, cook the brown rice according to package instructions.
- Toss the asparagus with olive oil, salt, and pepper, then roast it in the oven for about 10-12 minutes.
- Serve the salmon with brown rice and roasted asparagus.

Lysine/Arginine: 2595mg/1755mg

Shrimp Stir Fry with Vegetables

Ingredients:

100g shrimp (2150mg Lysine, 1280mg Arginine), 1 cup mixed stir-fry vegetables (e.g., broccoli, carrots, snap peas) (80mg Lysine, 100mg Arginine), 1 tablespoon soy sauce, 1 tablespoon vegetable oil.

Instructions:

- Heat the vegetable oil in a wok or large skillet over high heat.
- Add the shrimp and stir fry for 2-3 minutes until they turn pink and are cooked through.
- Add the mixed stir-fry vegetables and continue stir frying for another 2-3 minutes until they're crisp-tender.
- Drizzle the soy sauce over the stir fry and toss to coat the ingredients evenly.
- Remove from heat and serve immediately.

Lysine/Arginine: 2230mg/1380mg

Grilled Lamb Chops with Couscous and Grilled Zucchini

Ingredients:

2 lamb chops (3160mg Lysine, 1985mg Arginine), 1/2 cup cooked couscous (180mg Lysine, 180mg Arginine), 1 medium zucchini (60mg Lysine, 80mg Arginine), 1 tablespoon olive oil.

Instructions:

- Preheat the grill to medium-high heat.
- Brush the lamb chops with olive oil and season them with salt and pepper.
- Grill the lamb chops for about 3-4 minutes per side for medium-rare doneness.
- Meanwhile, cook the couscous according to package instructions.
- Slice the zucchini into thin strips and brush them with olive oil.
- Grill the zucchini strips for about 2 minutes per side until they're tender and have grill marks.
- Serve the grilled lamb chops with cooked couscous and grilled zucchini.

Lysine/Arginine: 3340mg/2245mg

Tofu Stir-Fry with Brown Rice

Ingredients:

150g firm tofu, cubed (1545mg Lysine, 1095mg Arginine), 1 cup mixed stir-fry vegetables (e.g., bell peppers, broccoli, carrots) (80mg Lysine, 100mg Arginine), 1/2 cup cooked brown rice (150mg Lysine, 150mg Arginine), 1 tablespoon soy sauce, 1 tablespoon sesame oil.

Instructions:

- Heat sesame oil in a large skillet or wok over medium heat.
- Add the cubed tofu and stir-fry for 5-7 minutes until it starts to brown.
- Add the mixed stir-fry vegetables and continue stir-frying for another 5 minutes until they're tender-crisp.
- Stir in the soy sauce and cook for an additional 1-2 minutes.
- Serve the tofu stir-fry over cooked brown rice.

Lysine/Arginine: 1775mg/1345mg

Baked Chicken Breast with Steamed Broccoli

Ingredients:

1 boneless, skinless chicken breast (4350mg Lysine, 2620mg Arginine), 1 cup steamed broccoli florets (70mg Lysine, 80mg Arginine), 1 tablespoon olive oil, lemon wedges for garnish.

Instructions:

- Preheat the oven to 375°F (190°C).
- Rub the chicken breast with olive oil and season it with salt, pepper, and your choice of herbs or spices.
- Place the chicken breast on a baking sheet and bake for 25-30 minutes until it's cooked through and no longer pink in the center.
- Steam the broccoli florets until they're tender-crisp.
- Serve the baked chicken breast with steamed broccoli. Garnish with lemon wedges.

Lysine/Arginine: 4420mg/2700mg

Salmon and Asparagus Foil Pack

Ingredients:

150g salmon fillet (4080mg Lysine, 1850mg Arginine), 8 asparagus spears (150mg Lysine, 180mg Arginine), 1 tablespoon lemon juice, 1 tablespoon olive oil, salt, and pepper.

Instructions:

- Preheat the oven to 400°F (200°C).
- Place the salmon fillet in the center of a piece of foil.
- Arrange the asparagus spears around the salmon.
- Drizzle the lemon juice and olive oil over the salmon and asparagus.
- Sprinkle with salt and pepper to taste.
- Fold the foil to create a sealed packet.
- Place the foil packet on a baking sheet and bake for 15-20 minutes until the salmon is cooked through and the asparagus is tender.
- Carefully open the foil packet and serve the salmon and asparagus together.

Lysine/Arginine: 4230mg/2030mg

Greek Salad with Grilled Chicken

Ingredients:

1 grilled chicken breast (4350mg Lysine, 2620mg Arginine), 1 cup mixed greens, 1/4 cup cherry tomatoes (10mg Lysine, 20mg Arginine), 1/4 cup cucumber slices (10mg Lysine, 20mg Arginine), 1/4 cup Kalamata olives (20mg Lysine, 20mg Arginine), 2 tablespoons crumbled feta cheese (100mg Lysine, 80mg Arginine), 1 tablespoon lemon juice, 1 tablespoon olive oil, salt, and pepper.

Instructions:

- Slice the grilled chicken breast into strips.
- In a bowl, combine the mixed greens, cherry tomatoes, cucumber slices, Kalamata olives, and crumbled feta cheese.
- Drizzle the lemon juice and olive oil over the salad.
- Season with salt and pepper to taste.
- Toss the salad to coat everything evenly.
- Arrange the grilled chicken strips on top of the salad.
- Serve the Greek salad with grilled chicken as a refreshing and nutritious meal.

Lysine/Arginine: 4490mg/2760mg

Lentil and Vegetable Curry

Ingredients:

1/2 cup cooked lentils (1565mg Lysine, 745mg Arginine), 1 cup mixed vegetables (e.g., bell peppers, cauliflower, carrots) (40mg Lysine, 60mg Arginine), 1/2 cup coconut milk, 1 tablespoon curry powder, 1 tablespoon olive oil, salt, and pepper.

Instructions:

- Heat olive oil in a skillet over medium heat.
- Add the mixed vegetables to the skillet and sauté for 5 minutes until they're slightly tender.
- Stir in the cooked lentils, coconut milk, and curry powder.
- Season with salt and pepper to taste.
- Simmer the mixture for 10-15 minutes, stirring occasionally, until the flavors are well combined.
- Serve the lentil and vegetable curry over cooked rice or quinoa.

Lysine/Arginine: 1605mg/805mg

Stuffed Bell Peppers with Ground Turkey

Ingredients:

2 bell peppers, halved and seeds removed (60mg Lysine, 60mg Arginine), 200g ground turkey (5130mg Lysine, 3240mg Arginine), 1/2 cup cooked quinoa (275mg Lysine, 275mg Arginine), 1/4 cup diced tomatoes (10mg Lysine, 20mg Arginine), 1/4 cup diced onion (10mg Lysine, 10mg Arginine), 1/4 cup shredded mozzarella cheese (100mg Lysine, 70mg Arginine), 1 tablespoon olive oil, salt, and pepper.

Instructions:

- Preheat the oven to 375°F (190°C).
- Place the bell pepper halves in a baking dish, cut side up.
- In a skillet, heat olive oil over medium heat and cook the ground turkey until it's browned and cooked through.
- Add the diced tomatoes and onions to the skillet and sauté for 3-4 minutes until they're softened.
- Stir in the cooked quinoa and season with salt and pepper.
- Spoon the turkey-quinoa mixture into the bell pepper halves.
- Sprinkle shredded mozzarella cheese on top of each stuffed bell pepper.
- Bake in the preheated oven for 25-30 minutes until the bell peppers are tender and the cheese is melted and golden.
- Remove from the oven and let them cool slightly before serving.

Lysine/Arginine: 5415mg/3480mg

Turkey and Vegetable Skewers

Ingredients:

200g turkey breast, cut into cubes (5130mg Lysine, 3240mg Arginine), 1 bell pepper, cut into chunks (30mg Lysine, 30mg Arginine), 1 zucchini, cut into thick slices (20mg Lysine, 30mg Arginine), 1 red onion, cut into chunks (10mg Lysine, 10mg Arginine), 2 tablespoons olive oil, 1 tablespoon lemon juice, 1 teaspoon dried oregano, salt, and pepper.

Instructions:

- Preheat the grill or broiler.
- In a bowl, combine olive oil, lemon juice, dried oregano, salt, and pepper to make the marinade.
- Thread the turkey cubes, bell pepper chunks, zucchini slices, and red onion chunks onto skewers.
- Place the skewers in a shallow dish and pour the marinade over them, making sure they're well coated.
- Let the skewers marinate for 15-20 minutes.
- Grill or broil the skewers for 8-10 minutes, turning occasionally, until the turkey is cooked through and the vegetables are tender.
- Remove from heat and serve the turkey and vegetable skewers hot.

Lysine/Arginine: 5190mg/3310mg

Lentil and Vegetable Curry

Ingredients:

1 cup cooked lentils (1600mg Lysine, 240mg Arginine), 1 cup diced mixed vegetables (e.g., carrots, peas, bell peppers) (40mg Lysine, 60mg Arginine), 1/2 cup diced tomatoes (20mg Lysine, 40mg Arginine), 1/2 cup coconut milk, 1 tablespoon curry powder, 1 teaspoon minced ginger, 1 teaspoon minced garlic, 1 tablespoon olive oil, salt, and pepper.

Instructions:

- Heat olive oil in a large pan over medium heat.
- Add the minced ginger and minced garlic to the pan and sauté for 1 minute until fragrant.
- Add the diced mixed vegetables to the pan and cook for 5-7 minutes until they're slightly softened.
- Stir in the diced tomatoes, cooked lentils, curry powder, coconut milk, salt, and pepper.
- Reduce the heat to low and simmer the curry for 10-15 minutes, allowing the flavors to meld together.

- Taste and adjust the seasoning if needed.
- Serve the lentil and vegetable curry hot over cooked rice or quinoa.

Lysine/Arginine: 1660mg/380mg

Quinoa Stuffed Bell Peppers

Ingredients:

4 bell peppers (any color), 1 cup cooked quinoa (550mg Lysine, 550mg Arginine), 1 cup diced vegetables (e.g., zucchini, carrots, corn) (40mg Lysine, 60mg Arginine), 1/2 cup black beans, rinsed and drained (260mg Lysine, 280mg Arginine), 1/4 cup diced tomatoes (10mg Lysine, 20mg Arginine), 1/4 cup shredded cheese (e.g., cheddar, mozzarella) (70mg Lysine, 70mg Arginine), 2 tablespoons chopped fresh cilantro, 1 tablespoon olive oil, 1/2 teaspoon cumin, salt, and pepper.

Instructions:

- Preheat the oven to 375°F (190°C).
- Cut off the tops of the bell peppers and remove the seeds and membranes.
- In a large bowl, combine the cooked quinoa, diced vegetables, black beans, diced tomatoes, shredded cheese, chopped fresh cilantro, olive oil, cumin, salt, and pepper.
- Stuff the bell peppers with the quinoa mixture.
- Place the stuffed bell peppers in a baking dish and cover with foil.
- Bake for 25-30 minutes until the peppers are tender and the filling is heated through.
- Remove the foil and bake for an additional 5 minutes to lightly brown the cheese on top.
- Remove from the oven and let them cool for a few minutes before serving.
- Serve the quinoa stuffed bell peppers as a delicious and nutritious main course.

Lysine/Arginine: 930mg/980mg

Turkey and Spinach Meatballs

Ingredients:

1 lb ground turkey (5150mg Lysine, 3585mg Arginine), 1 cup chopped spinach (30mg Lysine, 20mg Arginine), 1/4 cup grated Parmesan cheese (165mg Lysine, 140mg Arginine), 1/4 cup bread crumbs, 1/4 cup chopped fresh parsley, 1 egg, 2 cloves garlic, minced, 1/2 teaspoon dried oregano, 1/2 teaspoon salt, 1/4 teaspoon black pepper, olive oil (for cooking).

Instructions:

- In a large bowl, combine the ground turkey, chopped spinach, grated Parmesan cheese, bread crumbs, chopped fresh parsley, egg, minced garlic, dried oregano, salt, and black pepper.
- Mix everything together until well combined.
- Shape the mixture into meatballs of desired size.
- Heat olive oil in a skillet over medium heat.
- Add the meatballs to the skillet and cook for about 10 minutes, turning occasionally, until they're browned and cooked through.
- Remove from the skillet and let them rest for a few minutes before serving.
- Serve the turkey and spinach meatballs as a flavorful and protein-rich dish, either on their own or with a side of your choice.

Lysine/Arginine: 5480mg/3865mg

Salmon and Asparagus Foil Packets

Ingredients:

2 salmon fillets (4000mg Lysine, 5200mg Arginine), 1 bunch asparagus, trimmed (20mg Lysine, 40mg Arginine), 2 tablespoons lemon juice, 2 tablespoons olive oil, 2 cloves garlic, minced, 1/2 teaspoon dried dill, salt, and pepper.

Instructions:

- Preheat the oven to 375°F (190°C).
- Cut two large pieces of aluminum foil.
- Place a salmon fillet in the center of each piece of foil.
- Arrange the trimmed asparagus around the salmon.
- In a small bowl, whisk together the lemon juice, olive oil, minced garlic, dried dill, salt, and pepper to make the marinade.
- Drizzle the marinade over the salmon and asparagus.
- Fold the foil over the salmon and asparagus to create a packet, sealing it tightly.
- Place the foil packets on a baking sheet and bake for 15-20 minutes, or until the salmon is cooked to your desired doneness.
- Carefully open the foil packets and transfer the salmon and asparagus to plates.
- Serve the salmon and asparagus foil packets as a healthy and flavorful meal.

Lysine/Arginine: 4020mg/5260mg

Vegetable Stir-Fry

Ingredients:

1 cup mixed vegetables (e.g., broccoli, bell peppers, carrots, snap peas) (40mg Lysine, 60mg Arginine), 1/2 cup sliced mushrooms (20mg Lysine, 20mg Arginine), 1/2 cup sliced zucchini (10mg Lysine, 10mg Arginine), 1/4 cup sliced onions (10mg Lysine, 10mg Arginine), 2 cloves garlic, minced, 2 tablespoons soy sauce (low-sodium), 1 tablespoon sesame oil, 1 teaspoon grated ginger, 1/2 teaspoon cornstarch (optional, for thickening), sesame seeds (for garnish), cooked rice or noodles (for serving).

Instructions:

- Heat sesame oil in a large skillet or wok over medium-high heat.
- Add the sliced onions and minced garlic to the skillet and stir-fry for 1 minute until fragrant.
- Add the mixed vegetables, sliced mushrooms, and sliced zucchini to the skillet and stir-fry for 3-4 minutes until the vegetables are crisp-tender.
- In a small bowl, whisk together the soy sauce, grated ginger, and cornstarch (if using).
- Pour the sauce mixture over the vegetables and stir-fry for an additional 1-2 minutes until the sauce thickens slightly.
- Remove from heat and sprinkle with sesame seeds for garnish.
- Serve the vegetable stir-fry over cooked rice or noodles for a satisfying and nutritious meal.

Lysine/Arginine: 80mg/100mg

Snacks

Apple and Cottage Cheese Plate

Ingredients:

1 medium apple (57mg Lysine, 27mg Arginine), 100g cottage cheese (573mg Lysine, **188mg Arginine)**

Instructions:

- Slice the apple.
- Arrange the sliced apple and cottage cheese on a plate. Serve immediately.

Lysine/Arginine: 630mg/215mg

Pineapple and Ham Skewers

Ingredients:

100g ham (872mg Lysine, 713mg Arginine), 1 cup of pineapple chunks (21mg Lysine, 12mg Arginine)

Instructions:

- Preheat your grill or grill pan over medium heat.
- Thread the ham and pineapple chunks alternately onto skewers.
- Grill for 10-12 minutes, turning occasionally until the ham is heated through and the pineapple is caramelized.

Lysine/Arginine: 893mg/725mg

Soups

Chicken and Vegetable Soup

Ingredients:

100g chicken breast (2793mg Lysine, 1519mg Arginine), 2 cups of mixed vegetables (such as carrots, celery, and peas - average 200mg Lysine, 250mg Arginine), 1 liter of chicken broth.

Instructions:

- Cook the chicken breast and let it cool. Then, chop it into bite-sized pieces.
- In a large pot, bring the chicken broth to a boil.
- Add the chicken pieces and mixed vegetables.
- Lower the heat and simmer for about 30 minutes. Serve hot.

Lysine/Arginine: 2993mg/1769

Lentil Soup

Ingredients:

1 cup dried lentils, rinsed and drained (5820mg Lysine, 5920mg Arginine), 1 onion, chopped (10mg Lysine, 10mg Arginine), 2 carrots, diced (20mg Lysine, 20mg Arginine), 2 celery stalks, diced (10mg Lysine, 10mg Arginine), 2 cloves garlic, minced, 4 cups vegetable broth, 1 teaspoon ground cumin, 1/2 teaspoon paprika, salt and pepper to taste, fresh parsley (for garnish).

Instructions:

- In a large pot, heat olive oil over medium heat.
- Add the chopped onion, diced carrots, diced celery, and minced garlic to the pot and sauté for 5 minutes until the vegetables are softened.
- Add the dried lentils, vegetable broth, ground cumin, paprika, salt, and pepper to the pot.
- Bring the soup to a boil, then reduce the heat to low and simmer for about 30-40 minutes until the lentils are tender.
- Taste and adjust the seasoning if needed.
- Serve the lentil soup hot, garnished with fresh parsley.

Lysine/Arginine: 5870mg/5970mg

Disclaimer:

Remember to adjust the portion sizes according to your dietary needs. Always consult with a healthcare professional or a dietitian when making significant changes to your diet.